The Fountain Of Youth Tacos

Michael Kentros

Introduction

I did it! I managed to tip the scales at a solid 250 pounds at a height of 5'7 and at the age of 49. Divorced twice, just getting out of another relationship and being the proud owner of high blood pressure, sky-high cholesterol, pre-diabetic and huge hemorrhoids due to a diet of nothing but chemically and artificially flavored and processed foods, topped off perfectly by plenty of ice cold diet sodas. I had attained the proud status of being your average know-nothing American that the purveyors of death and illness, also known as the commercial food industries' favorite customer. The problem for the commercial food industry is that I was 49 and headed into a full-blown mid-life crisis, the like that would free me from their grip and allow me to witness firsthand the power and control one person can have over their own life, weight, health, looks and future.

Decided to head off to Greece and the Greek island of Zakynthos for the summer to get away from the disaster that was the life I had created for myself and to see the motherland I had heard so much about before getting any sicker or worse. I had received the results of my physical and blood work and after meeting with my doctor, I had heard all that I needed to hear for now. I packed all my fat clothes and headed off. While in Greece, I noticed something very strange. I was the fattest person in every room and place I walked into. Why weren't others as fat as me? What's going on here? I was never that fat guy in the room, or at least not the fattest. Oh well, huge red flag to the extent of what I did to myself. Next, I began to eat local food, fruits and vegetables, and this where the awakening or "ah ha" moment first came. Nothing, and I mean nothing, tasted like the food back home. It tasted, should I say...real. The vegetables and greens melted in your mouth like warm butter. The local meat tasted fresh, clean and pure but the diamonds in the ruff were the grapes on the vine and best of all, the figs bursting off the fig trees under the Aegean summer sun. They tasted as if they had been touched by the hand of God himself. The pears and peaches were almost as delicious as the sweetest candy you could ever imagine and I knew then what real food tasted like. In almost 50 years, I had never tasted real food but I was determined to taste it again somehow. Time came to leave the place with air so pure you can practically taste and the clearest water that helped sooth my beaten soul and off to America to begin the next chapter of a life that had been semi-wasted.

I was back in America coming to terms with the results of my blood work, physical well-being and meeting with my doctor who advised me that unless 75% of my plate was vegetables, I would be a full blown diabetic within a year. How on earth can I eat 75% vegetables? I'm a junk food addict! I love my pizza, cheeseburgers and hot chips, ice cream and popsicles. But I loved something else much more...life and my belief in myself that there is no way I'm going out like this. Hell No! I knew very little about cooking, let alone anything about organic, GMOs, artificial colors and flavors, but I learned quick. I knew I had to remove all these chemicals from my body if I stood a chance of beating this and coming back to life. I looked up healthy recipes and began experimenting with different dishes with my friend Chris and low! Behold everything we cooked tasted great and it was healthy and we were getting excited about this healthy lifestyle and the fact that we were getting away from processed foods. Then one day while I was driving, I found myself listening to news report that a national fast-food Mexican restaurant was accused of using only 30% meat in their tacos and the rest was fillers (any junk they can throw in to look and taste like food), then it hit me like a ton of bricks! What if I used only 30% meat in my tacos and the rest was vegetables? Then I would be doing what the doctor had advised, eating 75% vegetables. So I quickly went to work. I started by formulating the perfect food source that I could live by. Let me tell you; this was not an easy process. It took months to get the recipe just right. But then one day, it happened! The most amazing taste sensation to hit my palate since those figs straight from the trees in Greece. It was amazing! These tacos tasted absolutely phenomenal. I had everyone I know try them so I could determine if it was only me who found them so delicious, or were they really this good. Everyone and anyone who tried them was like, "OMG! These taste so delicious." People went just as crazy as I did. How can something that is practically all vegetables taste like a taco … but just not any taco, the most delicious taco ever? You may say that it cannot be done. Let me tell you; it can be DONE! And it's PHENOMENAL!

News Links

https://www.dailystar.co.uk/ diet-fitness/655660/How-to- lose-weight-fast-healthy-taco- recipes

http://www.dailymail.co.uk/ femail/article-5021895/Obese- man-s-life-transformed-taco- diet.html

https://nypost.com/2017/10/27/ teacher-finds-the-fountain-of- youth-in-tacos/

https://m.facebook.com/story.php?story_fbid=10155054793288441&id=107787018440

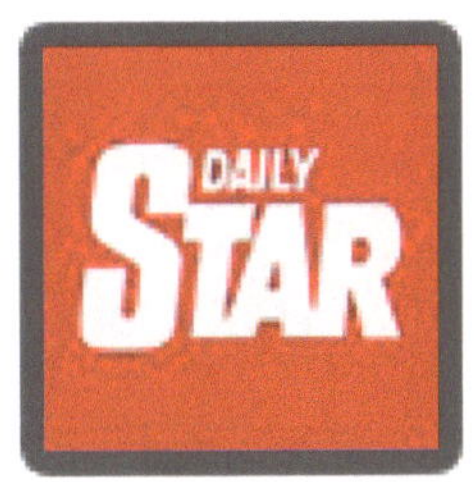

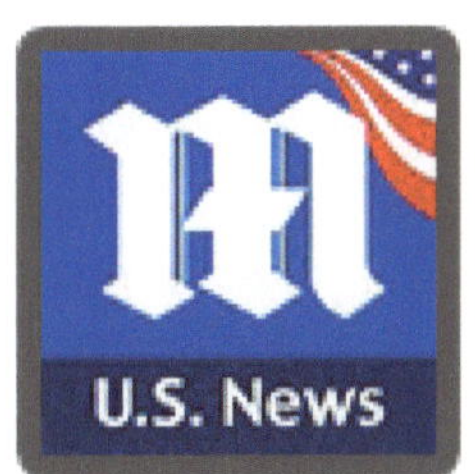

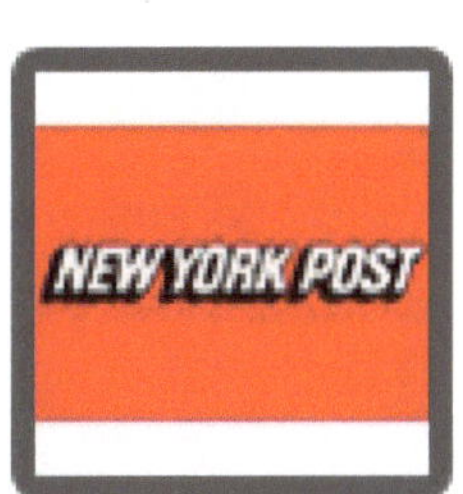

FINAL PRODUCT READY TO EAT

Enjoy in a taco shell, tostada or taco bowl.

This recipe batch is designed to feed 1 person for 4-5 days.

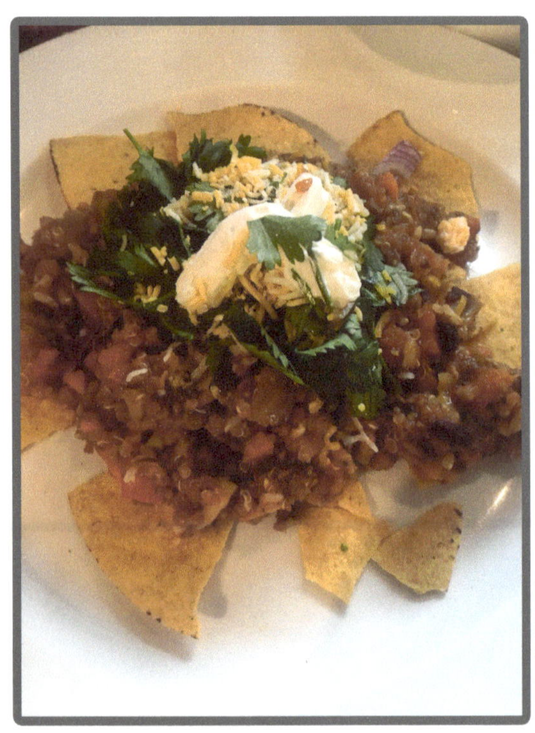

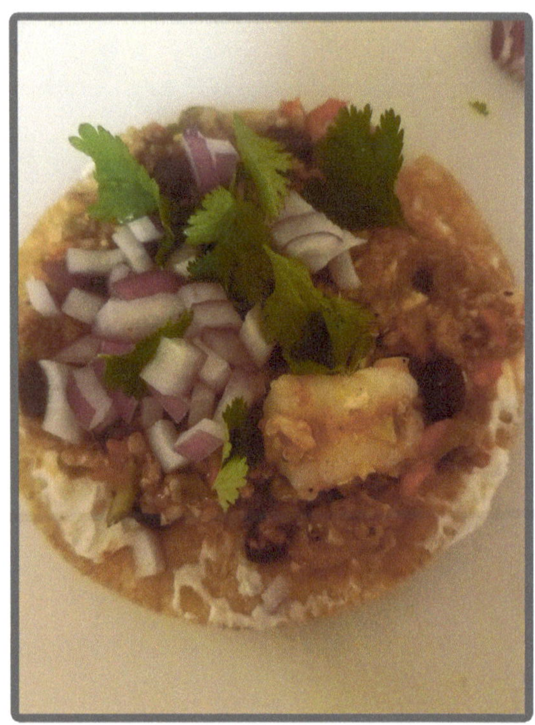

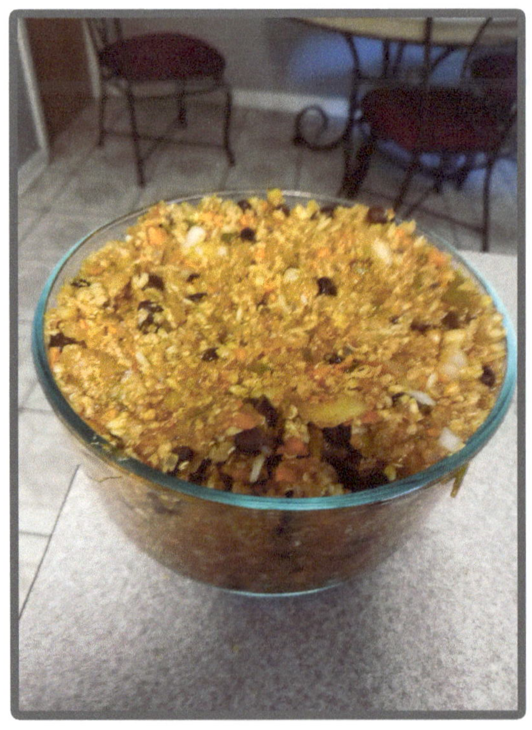

Taco Recipe

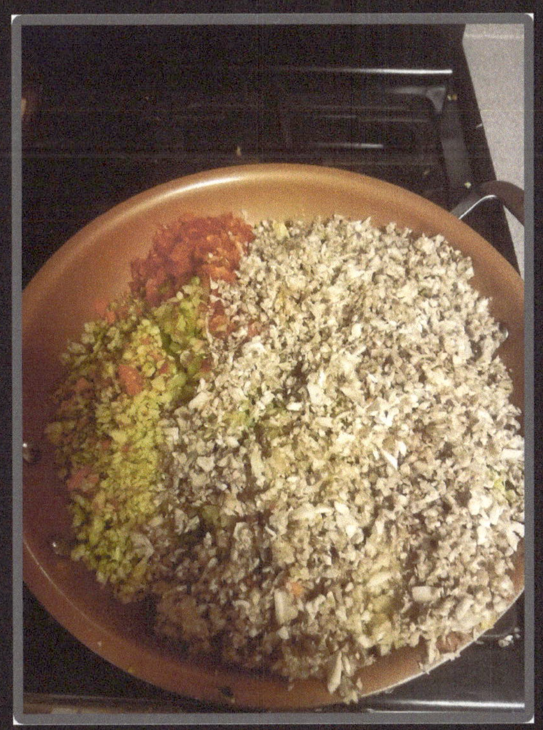

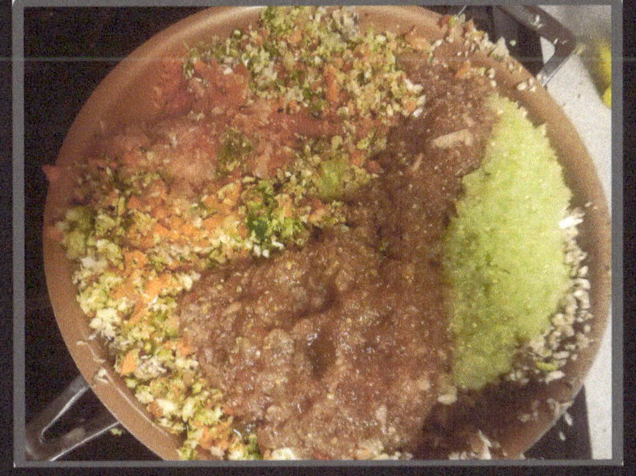

How To make?

Pour all ingredients after browning onions for a few minutes in 4 tablespoons olive oil.

Puree tomatoes and tomatillos in food processor and pour on top with tomato sauce

Let cook for a few minutes over medium flame. Then this is the point the magic happens. The spices will transform the vegetables into taco. And as we said before, not just any taco but the most amazing, tastiest taco to ever touch your lips while being the healthiest meal on the planet.
Add 5 tablespoons chili powder and 5 cumin. Take off the lid of spice jars and pour it out.
Add 1 big tablespoon paprika.
Add 1 tablespoon Cheyenne pepper, sprinkle very little oregano.
Add Himalayan pink salt and pepper to taste.

Walla! Taco is made! Continue to simmer till everything looks, smells, and tastes like taco...should take around 10 minutes for everything to come together. Let stand and drain excess juices.

Add the black beans and cooked quinoa/brown rice and blend. Let it cook for a few more minutes till the carrots lose crunch. This is your VEGETARIAN/VEGAN blend. It will taste amazing. It can stand on its own and you would never guess that there is No meat in it.

If you aren't ready to go full vegetarian just yet, not a problem. I lost all my weight in 6 months adding 3/4 pounds of 93% lean, ground turkey, grass fed beef or gulf shrimp to blend. It is so low in fats that the weight will shed off you regardless. bon appetite!

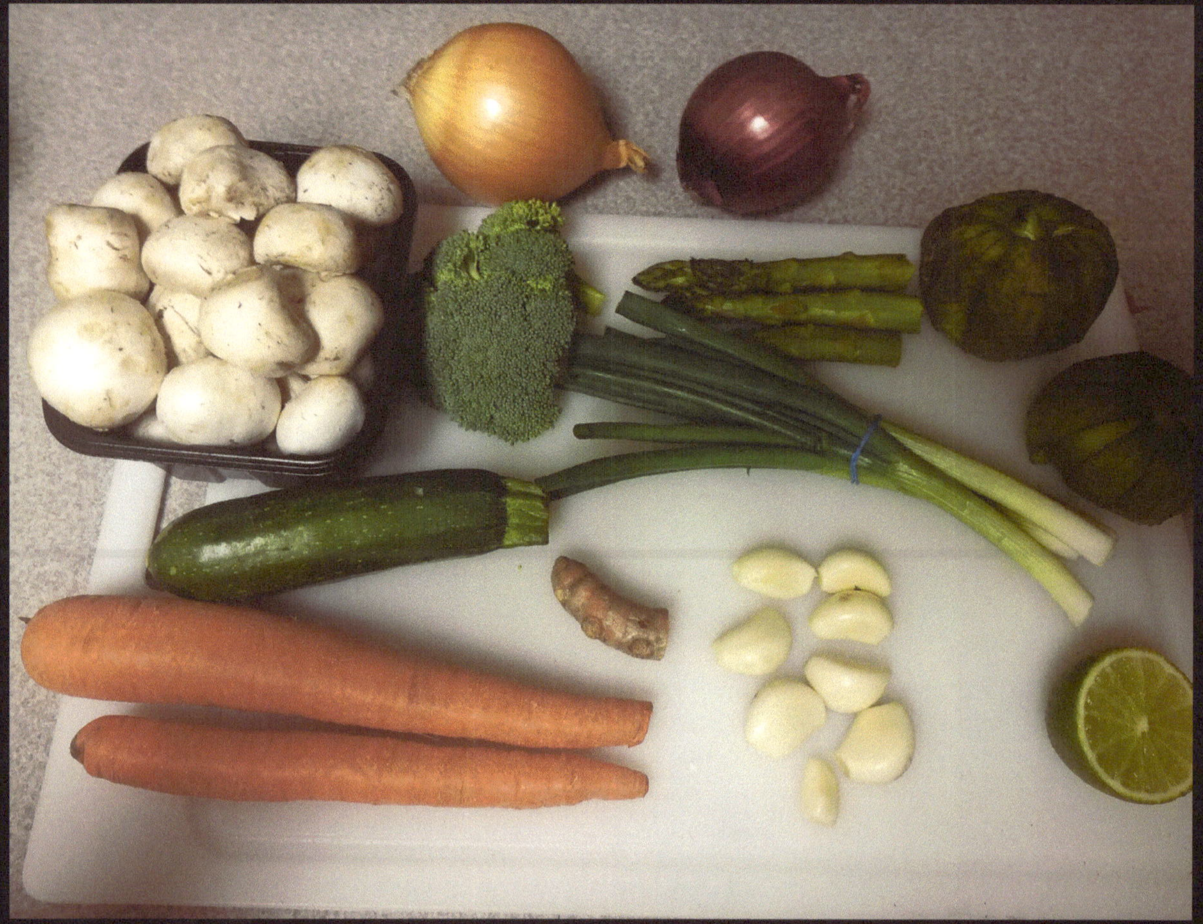

2 large carrots
6 large garlic cloves
4 green onion stalks
1 medium broccoli crown
8 to 10 thin asparagus stalks
1 medium zucchini
1 large red onion
1 med/large Spanish onion
12 oz. white or Bella mushrooms
2 large tomatillos
1.5-inch piece fresh turmeric
half lime

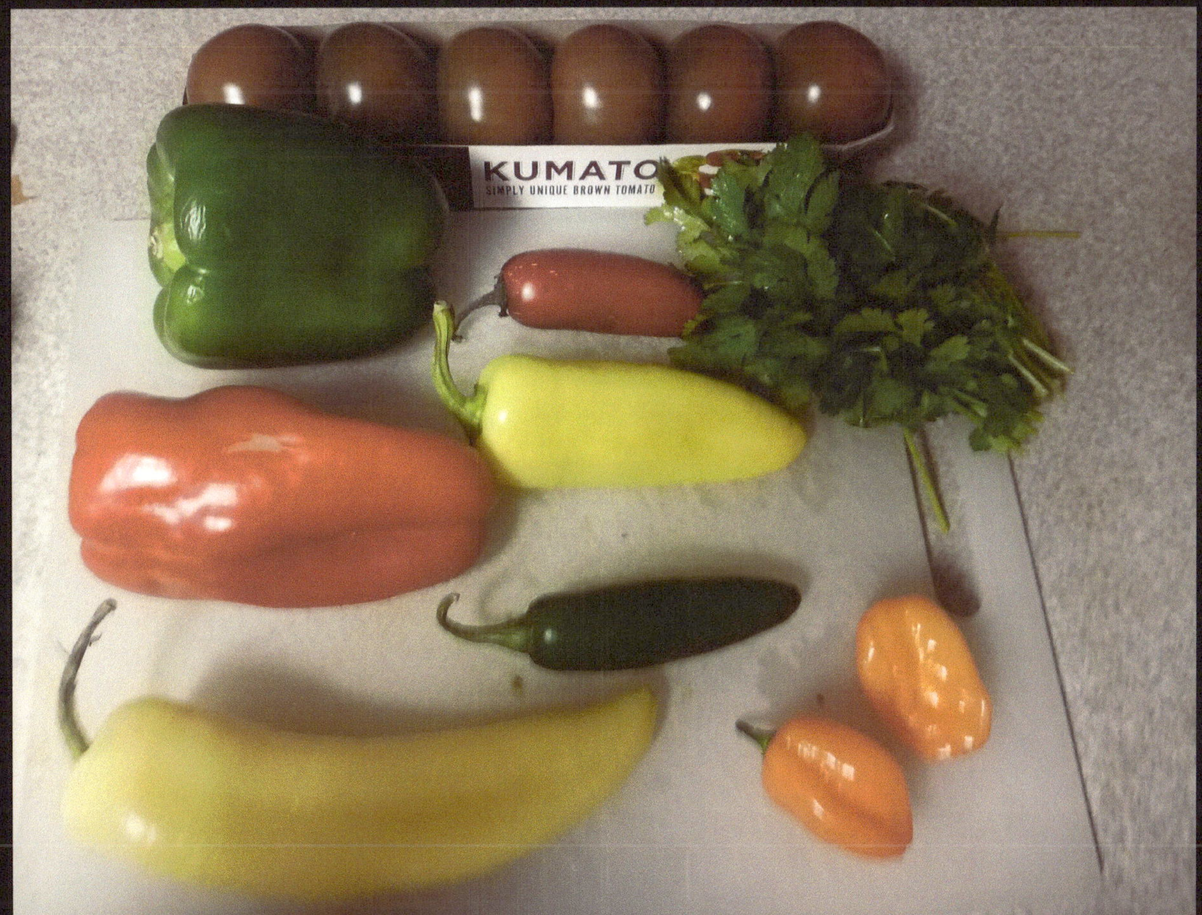

2 med bell peppers
2 jalapenos
2 banana peppers
2 med/lg habanero peppers
1 pound tomatoes
1 bunch cilantro
note: you may add a handful of spinach and Swiss chard but you should remove
either broccoli or asparagus to avoid any hint of greenery in taco blen

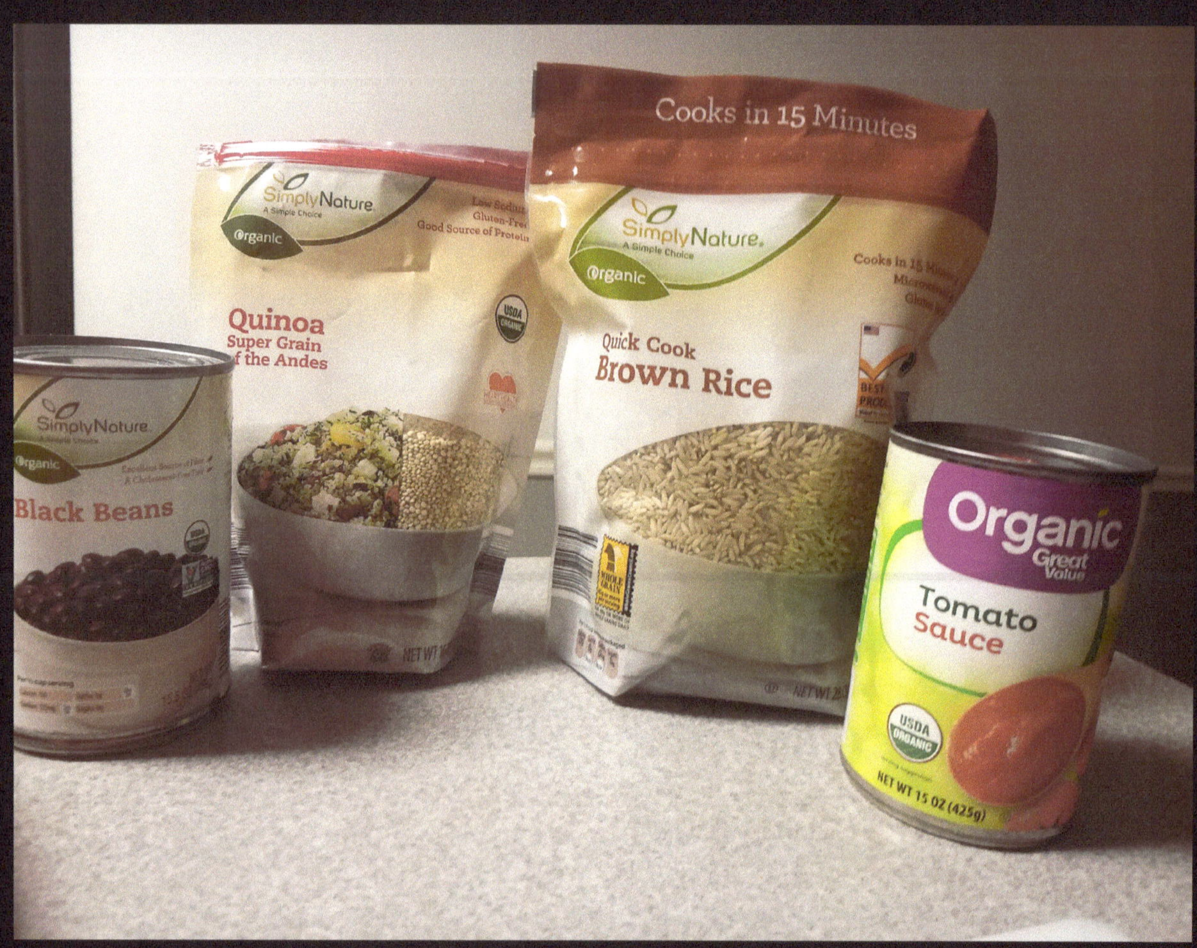

1 can black beans
8oz. tomomato sauce
quarter cup quinoa
quarter cup brown rice cooked together in a pot with 1 cup water. Rinse quinoa
before cooking

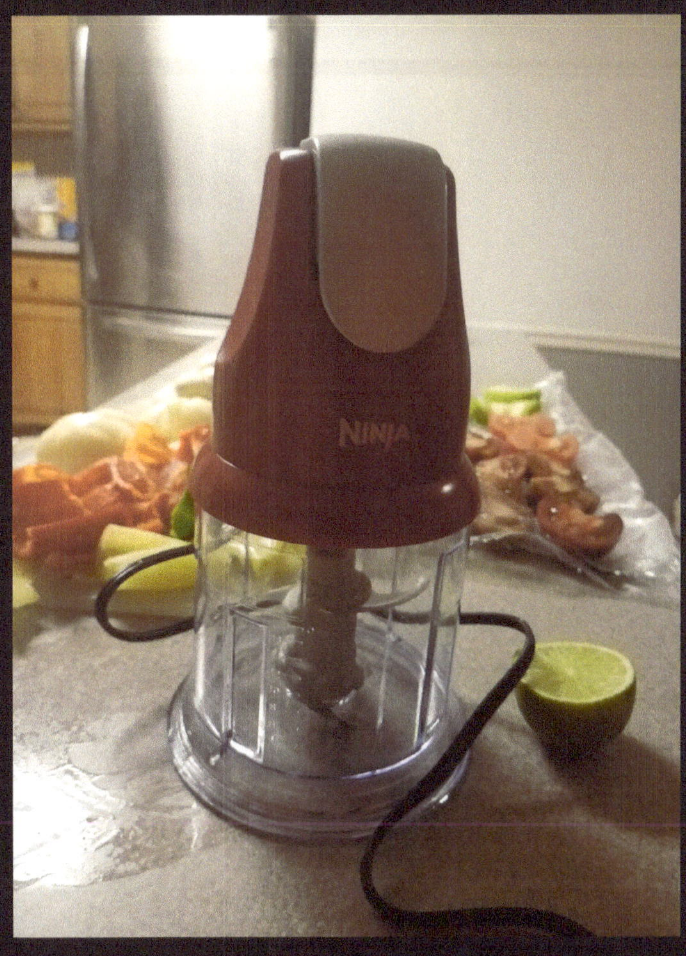

food processor to chop vegetables is a must!

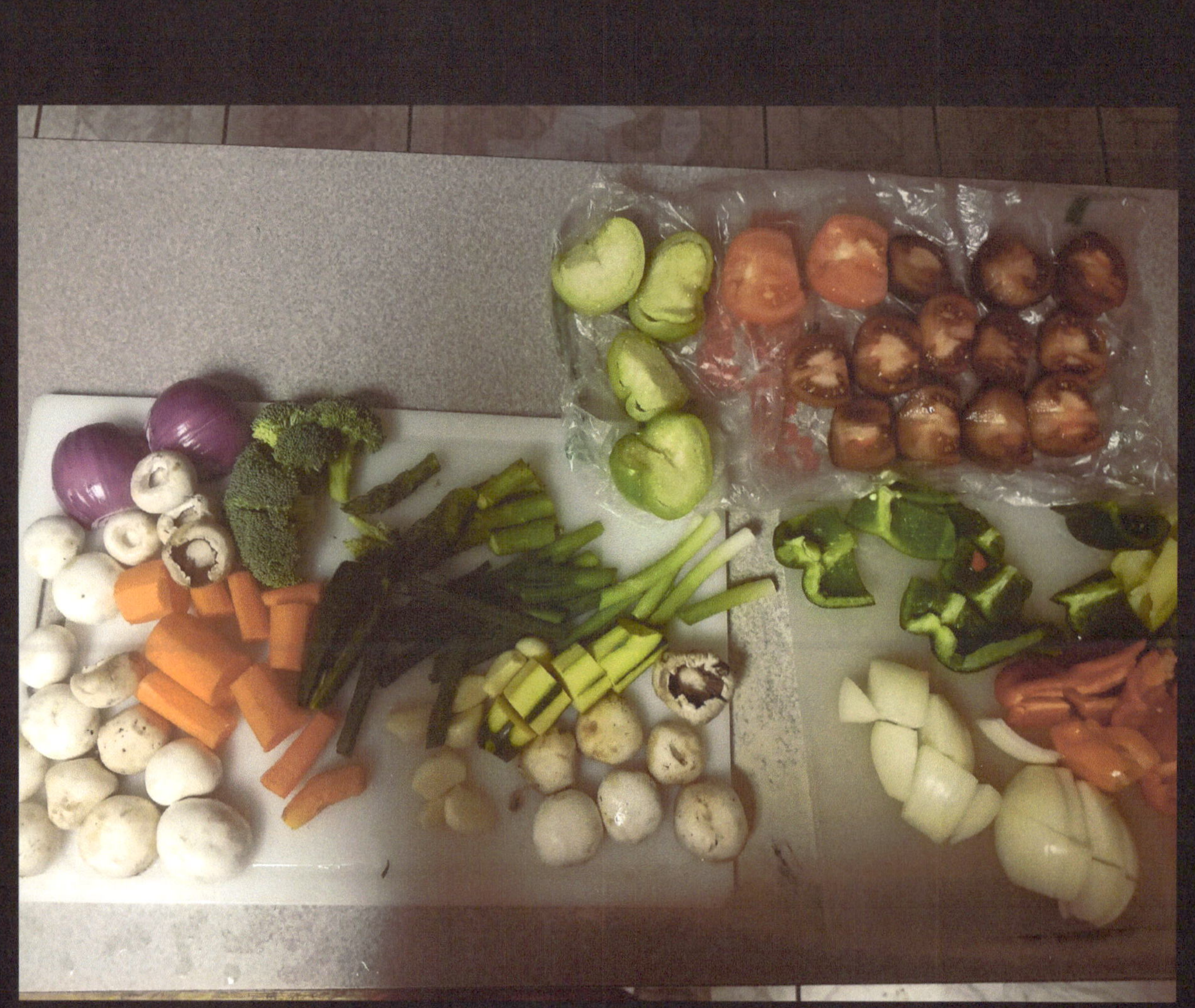

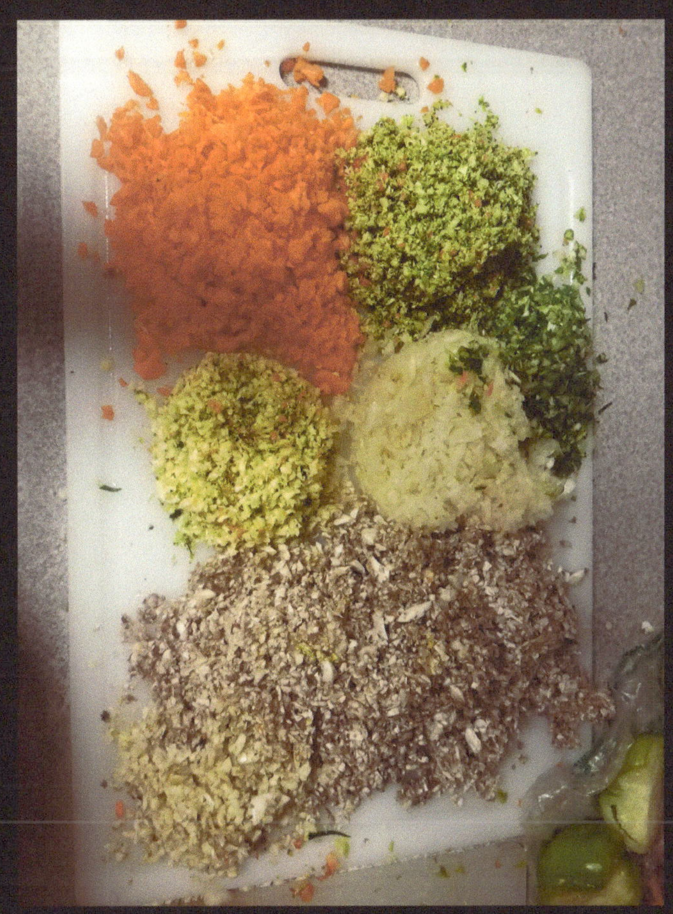

After chopping the veggies

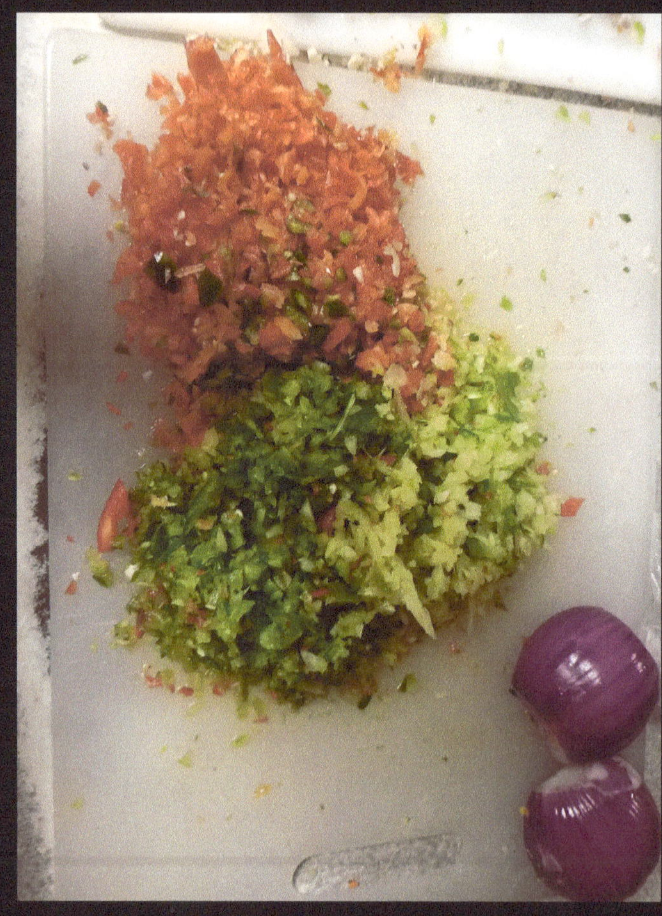

All the peppers chopped
Leave the red onion and cilantro for topping at the end

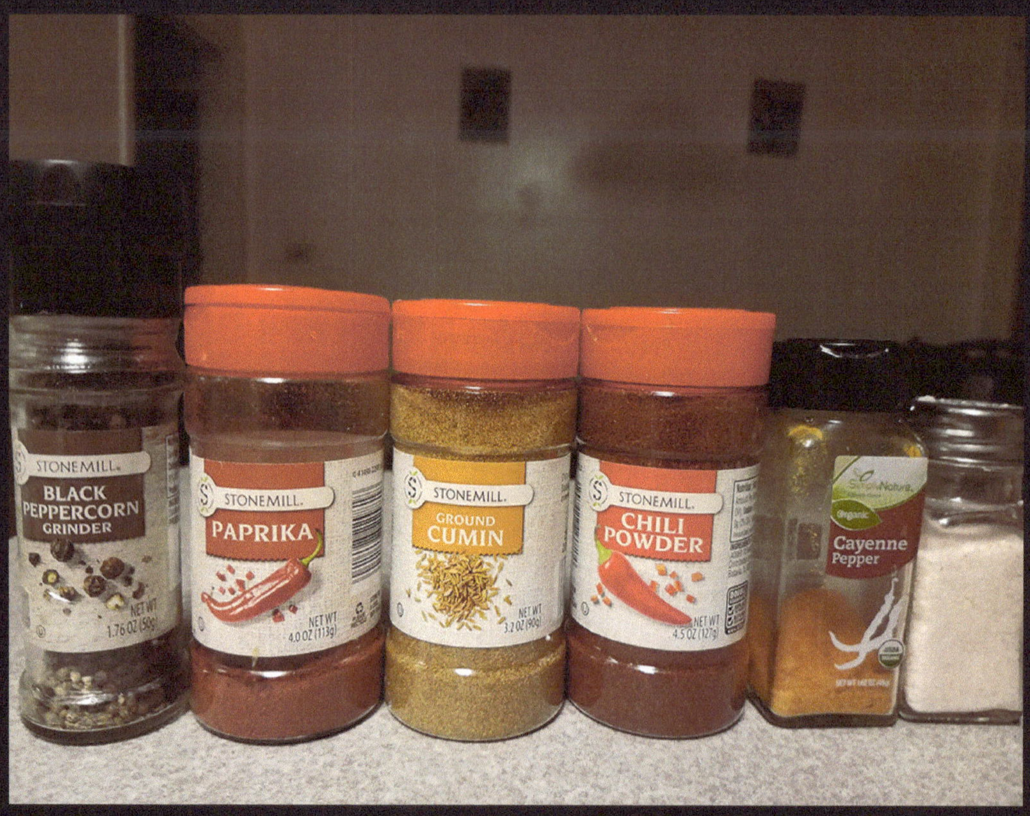

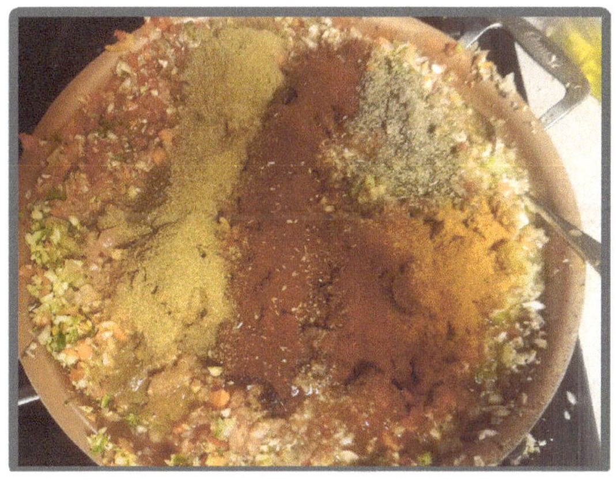
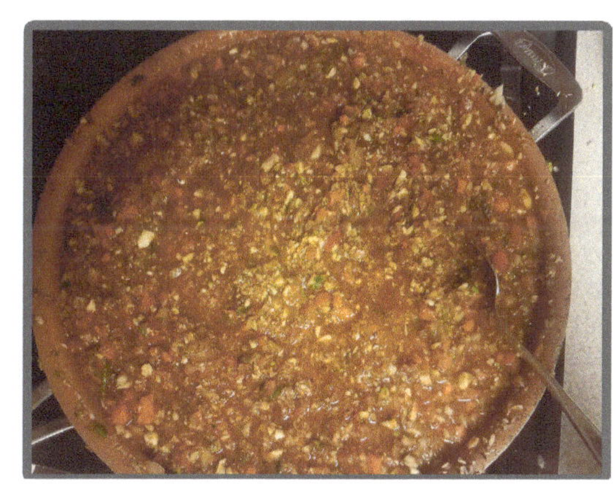
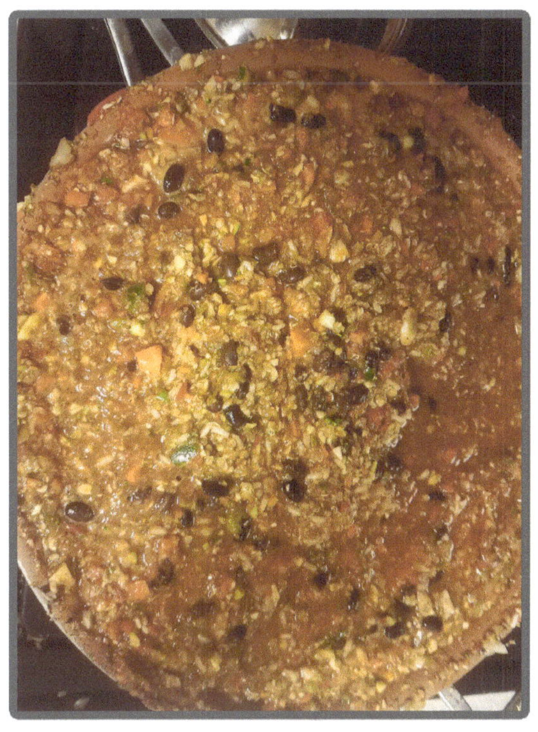
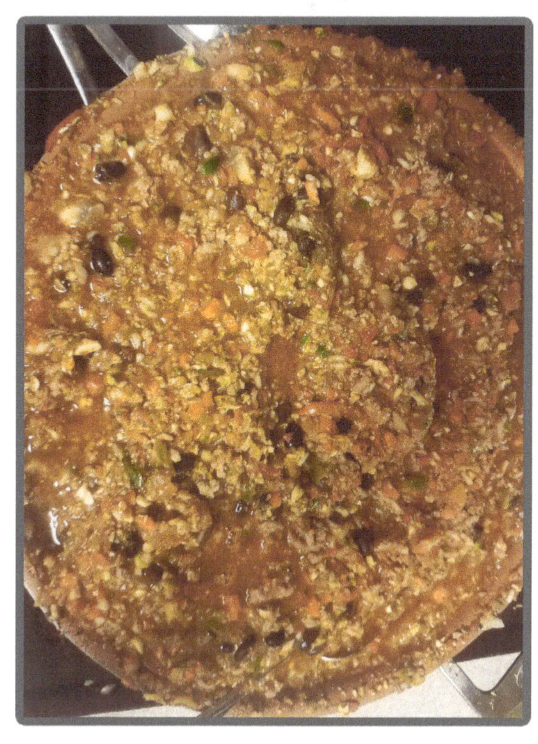

Fountain of Youth Taco Diet

What To Expect

You don't need to count calories ever again. Instead, start counting nutrients and you will be just as fine. This taco is more of a scientific formula than it is a recipe. An array of the most nutrient-laden and vitamin-rich vegetables (preferably organic whenever available) are combined to not only heal a damaged and sick body but also to renew it to its optimal functioning level while eliminating fats from your body. Don't be surprised if you are 50 years old and jumping fences again.

The specific vegetables were chosen because of the benefits each has for the body. It took so many vegetables to work on every system of the body, bringing health and vitality back to your cells, skin and muscles, basically turning back the hand of time ... sort of fountain of youth formula.

I believe this is the healthiest superfood on the planet. When you bombard your body day after day with these vitamins and nutrients, your body will have no choice but to respond in the most magnificent way. Keeping your liver from working overtime cleaning out junk allows your body to heal in many other areas, thus restoring you back to health and allowing you to ditch your meds for good.

After one week of eating healthy, most of your cravings will reduce. You will have more energy and find yourself doing physical activities you rarely did and your pants won't feel as tight.

After one month, your skin will restore the initial vitality. High blood pressure and cholesterol levels will start to drop. Your metabolism will increase and the weight will start to pour off after you enter your 2nd month.

After six months, you won't believe you were ever fat. You will feel great, look great and you will no longer be invisible. The opposite sex will show much more interest in you and you might find yourself getting tired of being hit on all the time becareful what you wish for. There is too much of a good thing ... but I will take that any day over the other option.

Congratulations on becoming a new person. Nothing about how you thought and saw things 6 months ago will apply to you anymore. You really are a whole new person. And I guarantee you will say, "I will never go back to the old me again." Have a happy, healthy wonderful life.

Get to Know Us

Everybody knows vegetables are good for human health but not too many people know why. A good exercise to do when deciding what food purchases to make is to ask yourself, or better yet ask Google, 'What are the benefits of eating ____ ?'

Getting to know your food and all the good or bad things it does for you is a great way to improve yourrelationship with it, or end it.
Let's try a few examples from our taco recipe:

Bella Mushrooms benefits - low fat, cholesterol-free and a rich source of essential vitamins and minerals that can enhance your health and prevent diseases. Nutrients include selenium, niacin, copper and pantothenic acid. Now, if you want to know what those nutrients actually do to your body, google them too. Knowing your food that intimately will ensure you will never take food for granted again and that you will always appreciate it.

Turmeric benefits - Increases antioxidants in your body, helps control diabetes, it prevents and treats cancer, as skin treatments, helps with depression, helps relieve arthritis and helps manage your weight. We love that one!

Onions - Improve immunity, they contain vitamins C and A, help reduce inflammation, helps prevent cancer, etc.

Carrots - Combats cancer, prevents cardiovascular problems, good for oral health, flushes out toxins from the liver, maintains healthy skin, aids in digestion, helps prevent stroke, regulates blood sugar and has anti-aging effects. We love that one too!

Garlic - Boosts immune system, reduces blood pressure, lowers bad cholesterol, promotes longevity, improves physical performance, detoxifies heavy metals from the body, keeps bones strong and aids in digestion.

Red Bell Peppers - Vitamin B6 and folate, packed with antioxidants, you burn more calories by eating them and helps improve night vision.

Zucchini - Source of antioxidants and Vitamin C, anti-inflammatory properties that improve heart health, very low in calories, a great source of energizing B vitamins and helps control diabetes.

Tomatoes - Antioxidants, a rich source of vitamins and minerals, protects the heart, improves vision, lowers hypertension, prevents urinary tract infections and gallstones.

Quinoa - High in fiber, Gluten-free, strong bones, high in protein, aids in weight loss, keeps the heart healthy, enables a healthy gut, and reduces the risk of diabetes.

This barely touches half the benefits of the Fountain of youth tacos but I wanted to give you an idea of how much punch this product carries and why it must be your main food source.

If you truly want to get thinner, healthier and younger-looking and improve your social/sex life dramatically, try this diet for 3 months. Remember you can still eat 20% junk and other foods. Just have taco as your main food source. Still hungry? Eat more taco. It's so low in calories you can eat all you want, up to 15 tacos a day. The only fat comes from a little sour cream you add and from the taco shell. So it's virtually free of calories.

Recipe 1

Don't forget to add a tablespoon of sour cream to your taco. We are on a diet not dead.

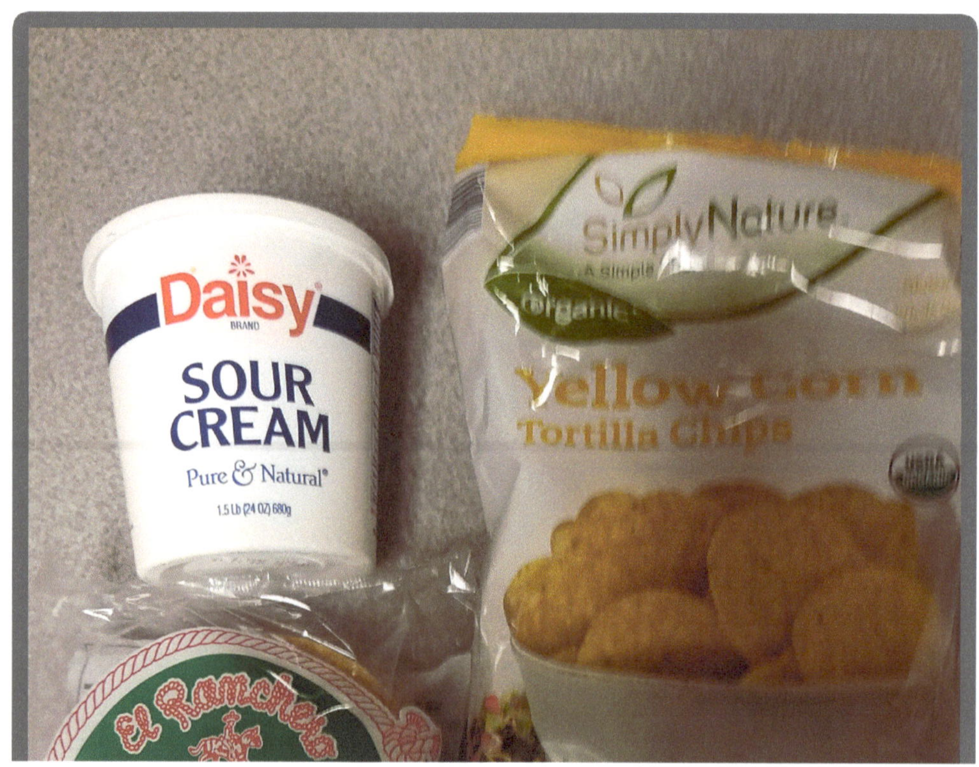

Recipe 2

I only buy el ranchero tostadas because they have only about 23 calories per tostada, other thicker ones have 60 calories each.

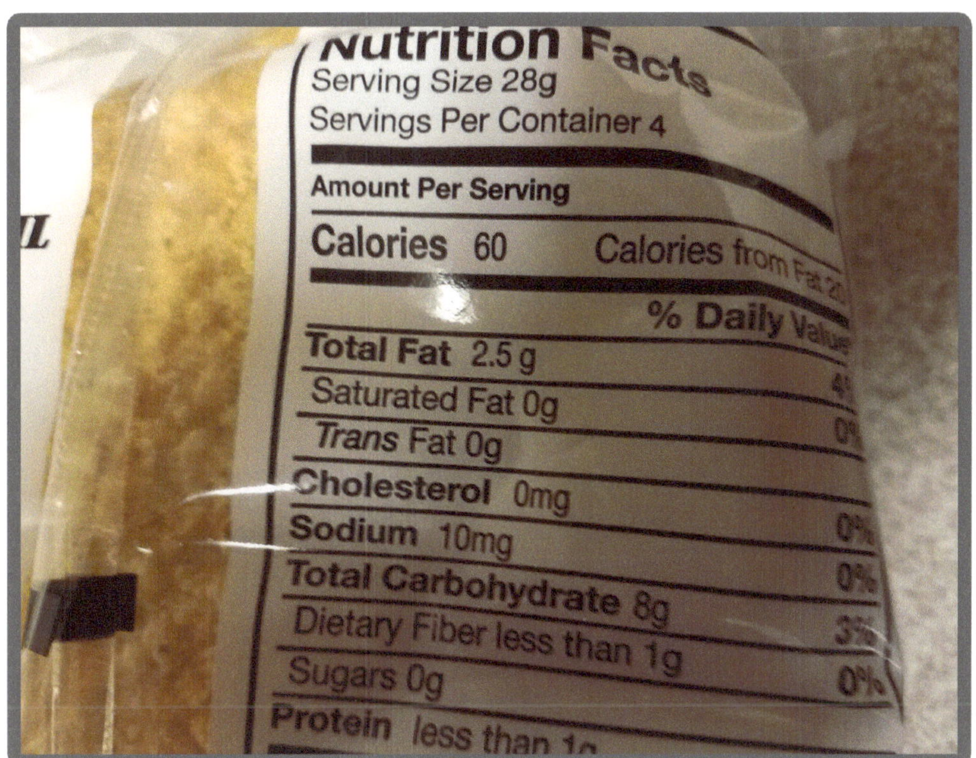

Taco Diet

People often ask me, "Don't you get sick of eating tacos all the time?" My answer is always quite simple. "Absolutely not!" I get sick of feeling sick when I don't eat tacos. Nothing out there is as delicious to me, as healthy for me and as enjoyable to me as tacos. If you are serious about losing weight, disciplined enough to make a weekly batch of taco and have it as your main food source, you are guaranteed to shed fat off your body. Just realize that you are about to go through something new in life to change yourself for the better and all the rewards you can imagine and have always desired will all be thrust upon you after a few months. You have to be sick and tired of being sick and fed up with being fat and unhealthy. If you are sick and tired and truly want to know what it is like to be young again and jumping fences, (yes I can actually jump fences again and so will you), then this is the easiest way to get there. Trust me; I am not a gym rat working the hardest rat maze to get to results.

Do you have to eat taco every day? No. Taco should be your main food source at the beginning. Eat as much as you want to fill you up while you slowly switch to 80% healthy 20% junk. This recipe is designed for 1 person, taken for 4-5 days along with other foods that you may want to snack on. I ate pizza and chips every week and still dropped tons of weight. Eat whatever you want but realize those choices may slow your outcome a little. Your desired outcome will come as long as you stick to tacos as your main source of food. Think of your body as a glass of water. If I toss in a couple teaspoons of dirt, it will still be relatively clean and clear. If I toss in a lot of dirt, it will be dark and filthy. Again 80/20 rule.

What else do I eat? I eat anything whole and real. Fruit, fish and seafood, roasted vegetables, soups and salads. Once you start eating tacos, your body will change. Cravings will go from weak to non-existent and when you happen to give in to your cravings, you will be like, "I can't believe I craved that, it tastes like crap now." All the foods you loved will taste disgusting once your body cleans up. You will be able to taste every fake ingredient in that junk. You will literally be given the power to taste chemicals disguised as food. Just remember to always use this and any power for good, not evil.

After 3 years on this taco journey and all the benefits I received from it, I have no other wish than to see others gain the same results and wellbeing from it. It truly feels amazing to look and feel young and healthy again.

michael kentros taco diet  

All   Images   News   Videos   Maps   More   Settings   Tools

About 241 results (0.58 seconds)

Obese Chicago man's life transformed by taco diet | Daily Mail Online
www.dailymail.co.uk/femail/article.../Obese-man-s-life-transformed-taco-diet.html
Oct 26, 2017 - **Taco** bout a quirky **diet**! Obese man, 52, sheds 50LBS by **eating** nothing but 12 **tacos** every day - and he says his trim new body has made him look 10 years younger AND boosted his sex life. ... Chicago substitute teacher **Michael Kentros**, 52, is hardly recognizable today thanks to his ...

Teacher claims the 'fountain of youth' is in tacos | New York Post
https://nypost.com/2017/10/27/teacher-finds-the-fountain-of-youth-in-tacos/ ▾
Oct 27, 2017 - A teacher claims to have found the "fountain of youth" thanks to an extreme **diet** which sees him eat almost nothing but **tacos**. ... **Kentros**, who is from Chicago, claims **tacos** helped him drop two shirt sizes and lose 50 pounds. ... **Kentros**, a substitute teacher at Chicago Public School ...

Teacher from Chicago, US loses 50lbs thanks to an extreme all-taco diet

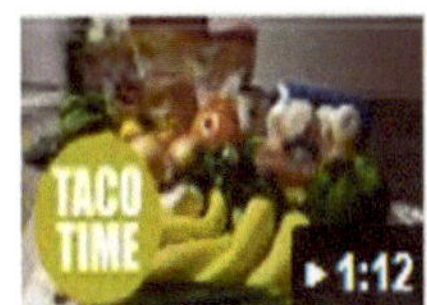

https://www.youtube.com/watch?v=4mAykiYZP7U
Oct 27, 2017 - Uploaded by SWNS TV
A teacher claims to have found the "fountain of youth" thanks to an extreme **diet** which sees him eat almost nothing ...

'I've never had this much action in my life': Man loses 3.5st by eating ...
https://www.dailystar.co.uk › Life & Style › Diet & Fitness ▾
Oct 28, 2017 - **Michael Kentros** claims to have found the "fountain of youth" thanks to an extreme **diet** where he eats nothing but **tacos**. The 52-year-old has lost 3.5st since switching to the new **diet** and says he looks ten years younger and that his sex life is "better than ever". Before he began to eat his taco diet, Michael's

The Project - An american teacher reckons his weight loss... | Facebook

https://www.facebook.com/TheProjectTV/posts/10155054793288441 ▾

I guess it would be irresponsible not to give it a try, right? Teacher claims the 'fountain of youth' is in **tacos**. A teacher claims to have found the "fountain of youth" thanks to an extreme **diet** which sees him eat almost nothing but **tacos**. **Michael Kentros**, 52, says he looks ten years younger, is 50 pounds ligh... nypost.com.

Obese Chicago man's life transformed by taco diet - WorldNews

https://article.wn.com/view/.../Obese_Chicago_mans_life_transformed_by_taco_diet/ ▾

Oct 27, 2017 - Two years ago **Michael Kentros**, 52, tipped scales at 250lbs and suffered major health problems. But he changed his life around by **eating** only veggie **tacos**, causing him to shed 50lbs. ...

Images for michael kentros taco diet

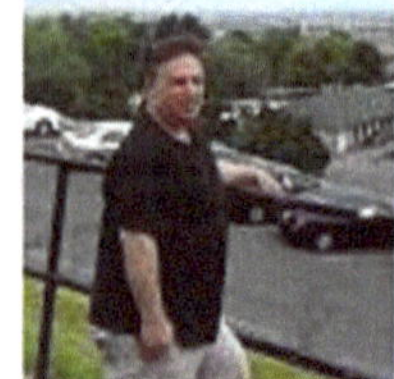 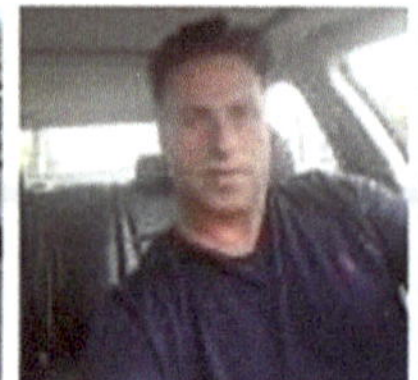 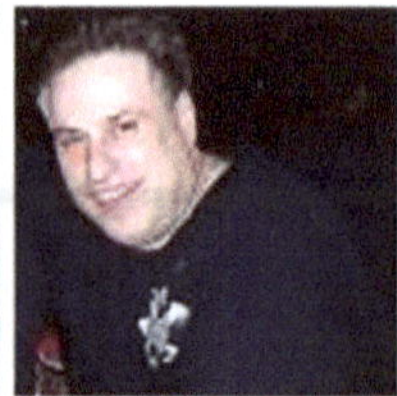 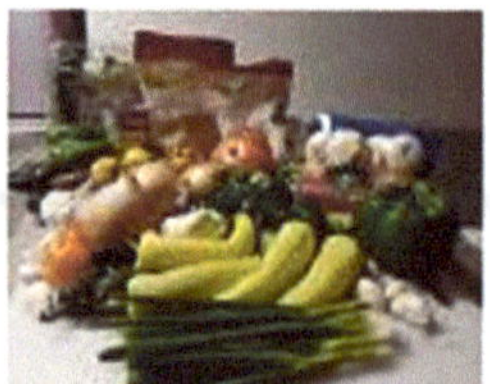 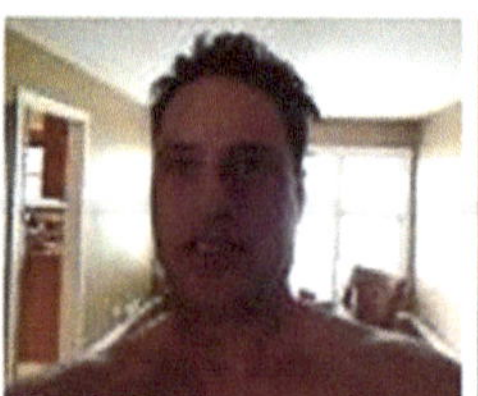 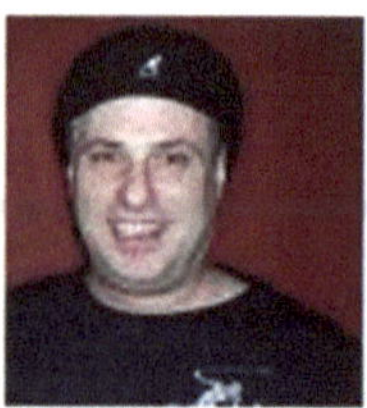

→ More images for michael kentros taco diet   Report images

Teacher finds the 'fountain of youth' in tacos - WorldNews

https://article.wn.com/.../teacher_finds_the_8216fountain_of_youth_8217_in_tacos/ ▾

Oct 27, 2017 - A teacher claims to have found the "fountain of youth" thanks to an extreme **diet** which sees him eat almost nothing but **tacos**. **Michael Kentros**, 52, says he looks ten years younger, is 50 pounds lighter and has a better sex life than ever since he began **eating** 12 homemade **tacos** a day. The former junk food ...

Chicago Teacher Loses 50 Lbs Thanks To An Extreme All-Taco Diet

https://rumble.com/v3vazt-teacher-from-chicago-us-loses-50lbs-thanks-to-an-extreme... ▾

CONCLUSION

Ironic we are in conclusion when it seems we have just begun. Now you have all the tools you need for your weight loss and a map to the fountain of youth. It will be a fascinating journey if you accept the challenge and I would like to make myself available for any support you may need along the way, respond to questions you may have as well as to be your greatest cheerleader. I am already at work with my cousin Evey, owner of Taco Junky in Colorado on new gourmet healthy recipes that will not only compliment the fountain of youth tacos but will also attempt to take them to a whole new level. Research and formulation of new exotic ingredients and recipes are ongoing and we hope to combine them into new superfoods that will launch your health and wellness into the stratosphere. Best of luck to all of you.